LOSE WEIGHT WITH LOW-CARB

George Calvert

ISBN-13: 978-1496035738

ISBN-10: 1496035739

TABLE OF CONTENTS

What Is A Low Carb Diet?   7

Benefits Of A Low Carb Diet   11

Are Low Carb Diets Safe?   13

Shopping Advice   15

Low Carb Diet When Eating Out   17

Maintaining A Low Carb Diet   19

Common Mistakes   21

Start Today   23

Chapter One

WHY ARE WE GETTING FAT?

O ne of the top health concerns today is weight gain and obesity. A leading causes of death today is obesity. Study after study has been conducted to try and find the reason for obesity.

Studies have shown that even though children engage in physical exercises, they still gain weight and in many cases become obese. For older folks, lack of exercise, has been found as one of the reasons for weight gain in addition to other factors.

In all of these studies, obesity and weight gain can be traced to the foods we eat. We have increased our food intake and we eat a higher percentage of sugar than we used to ingest about fifty years ago. The amount of fat that we eat has also increased. These two factors coupled with lack of exercise are the leading causes of weight gain.

The solution to these problems is to change our eating habits. One way of preventing weight gain is by starting a low carbohydrate diet. A low carb diet allows you to control the amount of calories you ingest.

The definition of a low carb diet differs depending on the amount of calories derived from carbohydrates or the percentage of carbs in the diet. Generally, a low carb diet can be defined as those diets that are between 5% to 45 % of calories from Carbohydrates. According to U.S. Government guidelines, calories from carbohydrates should be between 50% to 65%. Therefore, on a low carb diet one should limit the intake of foods with high carbohydrate levels.

The amount of carbohydrates that the body can tolerate varies from person to person. The goal is the reduction of the amount of carbohydrates taken in to levels that the body can tolerate. Mainly this means the reduction or elimination of foods from our diet like potatoes, white rice, white flour and sugar.

Weight loss is possible by the reduction of carbohydrates in our diet. Low carb diets should be closely monitored so that when signs of weight loss are noticed; the intake of carbohydrates is slowly increased until the body can control blood glucose.

The body should generate energy from fats instead of glucose. Energy from glucose diminishes quickly, while energy from fats improves stamina and is long lasting. This is known as the ketogenic diet.

WHAT IS A LOW CARB DIET?

We have probably heard about low carb diets and how effective they can be in losing weight, but what exactly is a low carb diet?

The term "low-carb" simply means low in carbohydrate. Carbohydrates are usually found in foods like pasta, potatoes, bread, pasta and rice. A low carb diet does not call for any specific diet nor does it include specific steps to losing weight.

It is a general term that varies from person to person. The consumption of carbohydrates causes the body to excrete insulin. A low carb diet then, include consuming foods that are low in carbohydrate and glycemic.

When we digest carbohydrates, our body excretes insulin which gets burned by our body if it we need immediate energy or gets stored as fat.

When we consume a meal that contains mainly carbohydrates, our insulin level goes up and goes down again after a short period of time. This causes us to be hungry again after only a couple of hours. This leads us to a circle of being hungry, then eating again. Consequently our body begins to store fat.

So, the initial question "What Is A Low Carb Diet?", depends upon whether you are talking about the actual carbohydrates consumed daily or the percentage of calories in a person's diet coming from carbohydrates.

As we said earlier, the normal amount of calories in an adult's diet is about 50-60%. So any percentage of calories from carbohydrates that is below that amount can be considered a low carb diet.

The main misconception about low carb diets is that most people on these diets actually strive to consume a zero amount of carbs. That is not only near to impossible, carbohydrates are in most of the food we consume, especially processed food.

A low carb diet as the name implies, is an attempt to reduce carbohydrates in a low level, not eliminate them completely.

Another myth is that on a low carb diet you cannot eat fruits and vegetables. This group of foods is rich in carbohydrate, but that doesn't mean that one should eliminate them from their diet. Fruits and vegetables are the type of carbohydrates one should consume in a diet that is low carb.

Some of the benefits from following a low carb diet, is first, the loss of weight and increased energy. People tend to be less tired and have better concentration and in some cases people's mood improves.

The benefits of low carb eating cannot be overstated. Individuals experience improvements in their metabolism, a benefit for a diet focused on losing weight. An increse in the metabolism is indispensable to a healthy way of life and weight loss.

Chapter Three

BENEFITS OF A LOW CARB DIET

When choosing a diet, you will want to receive plenty of positive benefits beyond losing weight. Crash diets or switching from one plan to another can actually be harmful. You should not focus solely on weight loss. You want to be healthier overall. You also should want to follow the plan for life instead of just a couple of weeks or months

By reducing the daily intake of carbs, some medical conditions you may be experiencing can occur less often or be illuminated. Headaches, joint pain, and trouble concentrating can be reduced. This may help you reduce the amount of pain medication you take.

Dieting can cause mood swings. The ups and downs of mood and energy can cause you to binge eat. Another plus for the low carb diet is balancing your mood and energy levels. The body gets more consistent energy from protein and other nutrients than it does from carbs. Carbs cause short energy spurts that will drop your energy level quickly after the carbs are digested. By lowering the amount of carbs you eat, your energy will come from other nutrients reducing swings in mood and energy.

If you exercise regularly to tone and build muscle, a low carb diet can help. After working out your muscles are sensitive to insulin. By eating a low carb diet, after a workout your muscles will draw in more amino acids from your meal. Amino acids help the muscles burn more fat.

Diabetics can benefit greatly from a low carp diet. If you have diabetes, a low carb diet can balance your insulin level. A low carb diet is a good healthy way to naturally balance your insulin and possibly prevent becoming a diabetic.

There are many benefits to a low carb diet in addition to just losing weight. You will have more energy and feel healthier.

Start eating more fruits, vegetables and nuts. Slowly reduce your intake of breads, sweets, and foods made from white flour and white sugar.

Chapter Four

Are Low Carb Diets Safe?

Obesity is one of the most popular health issues worldwide. It has received so much attention that the idea of weight loss has spawned thousands of business opportunities. The commercialization of this issue has had a negative impact on actual weight loss.

The two main variables in the area of weight loss are calorie intake and burning calories. They have been exaggerated so much that many weight loss programs are actually a threat to good health.

When your intake of calories drops the body begins using stored fat. This leads to weight loss. But will it be a safe process?

For example, reducing the fat intake without considering the type of fat being lost, might lead to elevated blood cholesterol levels. A properly designed diet would include polyunsaturated fats and mono-unsaturated fats which are considered safe.

The same theory applies to the nutrients. Some diets advise staying away from fruits and vegetables. These plans do more harm than good. Eliminating fruits like bananas and watermelon might be logical because of their high glycaemic. But limiting all the fruits and vegetables is bad advice where your health is concerned.

Reducing the intake of calcium rich food like whole grain could cause conditions like osteoporosis. Women with calcium deficiencies tend to suffer from menstrual issues. Most low carb diets advocate more on protein intake. Large amounts of protein makes the kidneys work harder. Proteins produce excess waste. An accumulation of harmful waste products can cause kidney stones.

Before selecting a diet plan a person should understand his or her own body. Kidney patient should pay attention to protein intake while a heart patient should concentrate more on eliminating fats. There are a number of factors that should be considered before following a low carb diet.

Lifestyle changes will require changes in your diet plans also. If you decide to start a bodybuilding routine for example, the energy demand on the body is different from what it was. In cases like these you should consult a professional.

Be careful with extremely "low carb" diets. They might not be safe. But a "correct carb" diet will give you the lean body you are looking for while being in good health.

Chapter Five

SHOPPING ADVICE

We know that packaged food is costly. Switch to home-cooked dishes made from tender meat and fresh vegetables. Pre-packaged junk foods will drain your wallet and it won't do any good to your waistline, either.

Consider purchasing fruits and vegetables when they are in season – that is when they are cheapest. It's also possible to spend less on meat. Expensive cuts of meat like beef tenderloin is a tasty cut of meat, chuck and sirloin cuts are delicious and cheaper in price. These cuts contain streaks of fat running through the meat, which makes them tender and juicy. Think about soups, stews and roasts. Purchasing a whole chicken and cutting it yourself will save you money.

Don't get into a rut. Break the monotony of your dinner meat by including something like eggs. They can be prepared in many ways like: poached, scrambled, omelette, quiche. Tofu and other soy foods could replace the usual sources of chicken and turkey protein, yet give you a variety of nutrients.

Make dishes that can serve as double recipes or as dinner one night and lunch the next day.

Have a plan. By planning your recipes and meals for the week, you won't be tempted to order take-out because you can't think of what to prepare for dinner.

Chapter Six

LOW CARB DIET WHEN EATING OUT

Worrying about what foods you should and shouldn't eat can be stressful. Eating out while dieting can be a challange. Eating out on a low carb diet is just the opposite. It is very easy to adapt food from almost any cuisine at any restaurant to fit your low carb diet.

Remember three things when dining out:

1. Know what you can eat, and what to avoid!
2. Plan ahead!
3. Stick to your guns!

Eating low carb gives you a lot of flexibility. Choices to look for when eating out include meat or fish that is not breaded or battered. Potatoes are off the menu, but why not try extra vegetables? If you want a juicy burger, have it without the bun. Salads give you unlimited options. Many restaurants offer different types of salad on their menu. Steak and mixed vegetables are a good choice.

The most overlooked part to eating low carb is planning ahead. By planning in advance, you'll already know what you can eat.

When eating out, stick to low carb. It is easy to be tempted by the bread basket, or by the desert tray. Don't give in to the pressure. Just remember, you deserve to feel healthy and be happy. There will be some foods you should not eat, but don't be afraid to ask for the ones you can.

Many restaurants are their menu items to accommodate dieters. There are lots of options available to you if you want to eat out. Knowing what you can eat, planning ahead, and sticking to it will keep you on track with your low carb diet.

Chapter Seven

Maintaining A Low Carb Diet

One advantage of a low-carb diet is that you won't have to worry about or keep track of the amount of calories you consume.

Maintaining a low carb lifestyle is all about the amount of carbohydrates in the food you are eating. With this type of diet, you need a plan that suggests the amount of carbs you take in everyday.

The idea is to decrease your carbohydrated and to reduce your sugar and insulin levels. Your body will begin to burn the stored fat in your body causing you lose weight.

Here are five suggestions to help you make the most out of your diet.

First, you need to have a checkup by your doctor. Consulting your physician is a good way to establish the best foods to include in your diet. The doctor will help you know what food to stay away from and what foods you should be eating.

Secondly, you must have an objective. The goal of any low carbohydrate diet is to lose weight. Setting your main goal will help you fit your diet into your lifestyle.

Thirdly, you need motivation if your plan is to work. Even when faced with temptations, stick to your goal. Imagine how you will feel and look when you reach goal.

Additionally, your attitude is important, be positive and believe you can achieve your weight loss goal.

It is a good idea to keep a journal where you can record your findings. This journal will help you find out whether your diet plan is succeeding or if you are getting off track.

Lastly, patience is necessary to eventually achieve your weight loss goal. Realize that it won't happen overnight but if you stick to your plan you will be successful. Maintaining a low carb diet, like any diet, is not easy. However, you will be successful if you stay with your plan and make it a habit. With time, it will become a lifestyle.

Like any dieting plan, you may get off track occasionally. It's not the end of the world. Simply get back up and continue with your plan.

Chapter Eight

COMMON MISTAKES

The following are the common mistakes about low cab diet.

Getting the wrong information - Some individuals believe that a low carb diet means eating meat every day. This is not true; you are simply trying to reduce carbohydrates in your diet.

Lack of sufficient fat - This happens as a result of thinking that low carb means low fat. At first, people can manage low fat dieting but this can lead to them using up their own body fat which means getting hungry very fast. It is important to add fat while on low carb diet.

Lack of enough vegetables in the diet - While on a low Carb diet, vegetables and fruits should be eaten in large quantities, especially fruits that are low in sugar.

Too much eating – Don't count calories in a low carb diet. Eat when you are hungry and stop when satisfied.

Poor planning – Eliminating old habits is not easy. If you fall off your diet, start again. It will take time for a new action to become a habit.

Use of low carb packaged foods - When buying low carb packaged food it is importance to read and understand the ingredients. Most packaged foods contain maltitol which is bad sugar.

Lack of variety - Most people might find the variety of foods available to them is limiting. The main thing to avoid in low cab diet is sugar **and starch.**

Insufficient fibre in the diet - Including vegetables and fruits in your diet will help to ensure that you are getting enough fibre.

Start Today

As we have learned, a low-carb diet limits the intake of starchy foods and sugar. A healthy amount of carbs in the diet give the body energy. The problem with an excessive intake of carbohydrates.

Tip #1

When shopping, pick the foods with a very low glycemic index; like apricots, apples, broccoli, asparagus, cauliflower, Brussels sprouts, green beans, celery, grapefruit, cucumber, cherries, mushrooms, lettuce, plums, onions, spinach, sweet peppers, strawberries, zucchini and tomatoes. Foods in the 'moderate-glycemic index' category are oranges, orange juice, grapes, cantaloupe, peas, peaches, yams, pineapple and watermelon. Stay away from the high-glycemic index foods such as raisins, potatoes, corn, carrots, beets and bananas.

Tip #2

Try low carb snacks such as walnuts, hard-boiled eggs, pecans, ricotta cheese. Go for the low-fat versions of dairy.

Tip #3

Eliminate foods that are high in carbohydrates such as pastries, soft drinks and potato chips. Remove all the rice, pasta, bread and grain products. If you can't live without bread, go for the whole-grain or whole-wheat variety.

Tip #4

Drink plenty of water. Water is not only important to keep you hydrated, but it also prevents cravings and constipation.

Tip #5

Read the labels carefully! This is a good way of controlling your portion size and carb-count of your daily diet.

Tip #6

Don't buy low-carbohydrate "alternatives" such as pre-packed energy bars or snack bars.

Remember, if you want your diet to work you must plan it properly first and stick with it. Start now and drop the fat the low carb way.